# WEIGHT LOSS & ENCOURAGEMENT QUOTES

## Health Quotes & Sayings

## Fun, Facts & Quotes

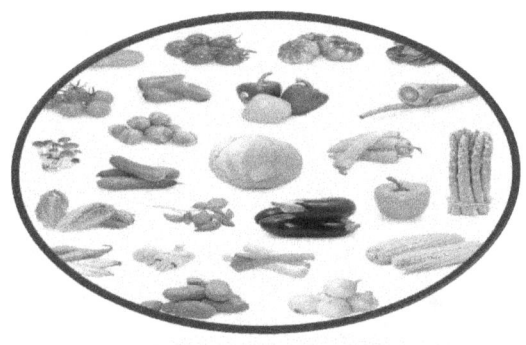

Compiled by Timothy Jonah

**Introduction:**

This mini book contain powerful nuggets and tips in the sayings which do have far reaching and positive inspiring effect on the reader; no matter your profession, age or sphere.

Tips and sayings that relates to your:

- ❖ Body, exercising, healthy eating and shape keeping
- ❖ Health and wellness
- ❖ Living in a mentally, socially; family and psychological balanced life
- ❖ Discipline, encouragement, motivation and persistency!

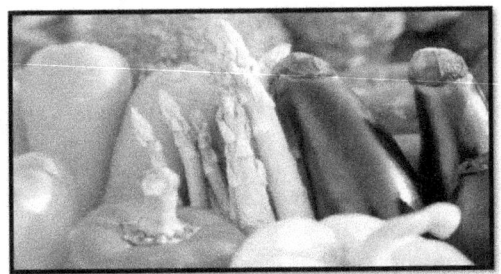

1. 90% of resistance is cautionary. - Shigeo Shingo
2. A big shot is a little shot that keeps shooting. - Anonymous
3. A change from unhealthy habits to healthy habits will yield extraordinary results. – Anonymous
4. A cheerful heart is good medicine, but a crushed spirit dries up the bones. - Proverbs 17:22
5. A diet is when you watch what you eat and wish you could eat what you watch. - Hermione Gingold
6. A fit, healthy body—that is the best fashion statement - Jess C. Scott
7. A good laugh and a long sleep are the best cures in the doctor's book. - Irish Proverb
8. A healthy body is a guest-chamber for the soul; a sick body is a prison. - Francis Bacon
9. A man should look for what is, and not for what he thinks should be. - Albert Einstein
10. A man who views the world the same at fifty as he did at twenty has wasted thirty years of his life. - Muhammad Ali
11. A merry heart does good, like medicine, But a broken spirit dries the bones Proverbs 17:22
12. A peaceful heart leads to a healthy body; jealousy is like cancer in the bones. - Proverbs 14:30

13. A person who never made a mistake never tried anything new. - Albert Einstein
14. A pessimist is one who makes difficulties of his opportunities, and an optimist is one who makes opportunities of his difficulties. - Harry Truman
15. A sound mind in a sound body is a thing to be prayed for. – Juvenal

16. A strong woman knows she has strength for the journey, but a woman of strength knows that it is within the journey she will find her strength. – C. J. Lewis

17. A wise man ought to realize that health is his most valuable possession. - Hippocrates
18. A woman's health is her capital. - Harriet Beecher Stowe

19. A year from now, you may wish you had started today- Robert Schuller

20. A young man with good health and a poor appetite can save up money. - James Montgomery Bailey

21. Accomplishment of small things leads to mighty things... - C. Hardy

22. Adversity reveals genius, prosperity conceals it. Horace

23. After a lifetime of losing and gaining weight, I get it. No matter how you slice it, weight loss comes down to the simple formula of calories in, calories out. - Valerie Bertinelli
24. After dinner, rest awhile, after supper, walk a mile. - Arabic Proverb

25. An idea can turn to dust or magic, depending on the talent that rubs against it. - Bill Bernbach

26. An ounce of prevention is worth a pound of cure. - Ben Franklin

27. "And put a knife to your throat if you are a man given to appetite." - Proverbs 23:2

28. And I think of that again as I've written in several of my beauty books, a lot of health comes from the proper eating habits, which are something that – you know, I come from generation that wasn't – didn't have a lot of food. – Joan Collins

29. Always be a first-rate version of yourself, instead of a second-rate version of somebodyelse . – Judy Garland

30. Another good reducing exercise consists in placing both hands against the table edge and pushing back. – Robert Quillen

31. Anyone can become angry---that is easy.? But to be angry with the right person, to the right degree, at the right time, for the right purpose, and in the right way---this is not easy. – Aristotle

32. Anything is possible. You can be told that you have a 90-percent chance or a 50-percent chance or a 1- percent chance, but you have to believe, and you have to fight. - Lance Armstrong

33. Appearance of a disease is swift as an arrow; its disappearance slow, like a thread. - Chinese Proverb

34. Associated with this weight gain are increased risks in adulthood for joint problems, angina, high blood pressure, heart attacks, strokes, type 2 diabetes and, ultimately, premature death. Outside of the human costs, health experts estimate that treating adult obesity-related ailments will cost the American economy nearly $150 billion in 2009. - Jeff Schweitzer

35. Be sober and temperate, and you will be healthy. Be in general virtuous and you will be happy. - Benjamin Franklin
36. Be the change you want to see in the world. - Mohandas Gandhi
37. Being defeated is often a temporary condition. Giving up is what makes it permanent. - Marilyn Vos Savant
38. Beauty is not in the face; beauty is a light in the heart. - Kahlil Gibran

39. "But I discipline my body and bring it into subjection..."- Corinthians 9:27

40. Challenges are gifts that force us to search for a new center of gravity. Don't fight them. Just find a different way to stand. – Oprah Winfrey

41. Cheerfulness is the best promoter of health and is as friendly to the mind as to the body. - Joseph Addison
42. Choose to be up here at the top, not down there at the bottom. - Anonymous
43. Clear your mind of can't. - Dr. Samuel Johnson
44. Coming together is a beginning. Keeping together is progress. Working together is success. - Henry Ford

45. Complaining will not change things in your life; only action will. Make a list of all you need to do to change what doesn't work in your life and, little by little, begin making those changes. - Susan Jeffers

46. Courage doesn't mean you don't get afraid. Courage means you don't let fear stop you. - Bethany Hamilton
47. Courage is what it takes to stand up and speak, Courage is also what it takes to sit down and listen. - Sir Winston Churchill

48. Creativity is a type of learning process where the teacher and pupil are located in the same individual. - Arthur Koestler

49. Cutting back on calories is not the answer to successful weight loss and successful health... you have to increase the quality of what you eat, not just reduce the quantity. - Joel Fuhrman

50. Diseases are penalties we pay for overindulgence, or for our neglect of the means of health. - Bulwer

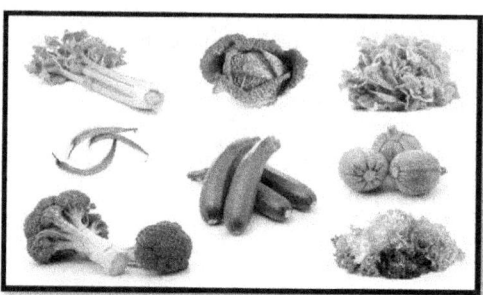

51. Diseases of the soul are more dangerous and more numerous than those of the body. - Cicero

52. Do not think of today's failures, but of the success that may come tomorrow. You have set yourself a difficult task, but you will succeed if you persevere; and you will find a joy in overcoming obstacles. – Helen Keller

53. Do the best you can in every task, no matter how unimportant it may seem at the time. No one learns more about a problem than the person at the bottom. – Sandra DayO'Connor

54. Don't ask yourself what the world needs. Ask yourself what makes you come alive, and go do that, because what the world needs is people who have come alive. - Gil Bailie

55. Don't be impressed with your own wisdom. Instead, fear the LORD and turn away from evil. Then you will have healing for your body and strength for your bones. - Proverbs 3:7-8

56. Don't dwell on what went wrong. Instead, focus on what to do next. Spend your energies on moving forward toward finding the answer. - Denis Waitley

57. Don't give up what you want most in swap for what you want right now – Anomymous

58. Don't wait until everything is just right. It will never be perfect. There will always be challenges, obstacles and less than perfect conditions. So what? Get started now. With each step you take, you will grow stronger, more and more skilled, more and more self-confident and more and more successful. – Mark Victor Hansen

59. Eat clean. Drink water. Stay active. Be healthy. – Anonymous

60. Eat like a pig and you will look like one. - Daniel L. Worona

61. Eat less, taste more. - Chinese Proverb

62. Eat not to dullness, drink not to elevation. - Benjamin Franklin

63. Eat to live, and not live to eat. - Ben Franklin

64. Eating crappy food isn't a reward -- it's a punishment. — Drew Carey

65. Eating healthy nutritious food is the simple and right solution to get rid of excess body weight effortlessly and become slim and healthy forever. - Subodh Gupta

66. Eating everything you want is not that much fun. When you live a life with no boundaries, there's less joy. If you can eat anything you want to, what's the fun in eating anything you want to? - Tom Hanks

67. Education is not a product: mark, diploma, job, money in that order; it is a process, a never ending one. Bel Kaufman

68. Even if conventional medicine tells you that your condition is incurable or that your only option is to live a life dependent on drugs with troublesome side effects, there is hope for improving or reversing your condition. - Leon Chaitow

69. Every accomplishment starts with the decision to try. – Gail Devers

70. Every human being is the author of his own health or disease. - Sivananda

71. Every time you are tempted to react in the same old way, ask if you want to be a prisoner of the past or a pioneer of the future. - Deepak Chopra

72. Every weight loss program, no matter how positively it's packaged, whispers to you that you're not right. You're not good enough. You're unacceptable and you need to be fixed. — Kim Brittingham

73. Excellence is not an act but a habit. - Aristotle

74. Excess exercise tends to be counterbalanced by excess hunger, exemplified by the phrase 'working up an appetite.' A few people with extraordinary willpower can resist such hunger day after day, but for the vast majority, weight loss through exercise is a flawed option. - Andrew Weil

75. Failure is not fatal; failing to change will be. - John Wooden

76. Failure is the mother of success. - Chinese Proverb

77. Failure is the opportunity to begin again more intelligently - Henry Ford

78. Fall seven times, stand up eight times. - Japanese Proverb

79. Focus on where you want to go, not on what you fear. - Anthony Robbins

80. Food is an important part of a balanced diet. - Fran Lebowitz

81. For a righteous man may fall seven times And rise again, But the wicked shall fall by calamity. – Proverbs 24:16

82. For most celebrities, the biggest meal of the day is toothpaste (they use reduced-fat Crest). - Dave Barry

83. For want of a nail a shoe was lost," for want of a shoe a horse was lost," for want of a horse a rider was lost," for want of a rider an army was lost," for want of an army a battle was lost," for want of a battle the war was lost," for want of the war the kingdom was lost, " and all for the want of a little horseshoe nail. – Benjamin Franklin's Root Cause Analysis

84. For whatever reason, maybe it's because of my story, but people associate Livestrong with exercise and physical fitness, health and lifestyle choices like that. – Lance Armstrong

85. From the bitterness of disease man learns the sweetness of health. - Anonymous

86. Give me a dozen heartbreaks...if you think it would help me lose one pound. – Colette

87. Give me a stock clerk with a goal and I'll give you a man who will make history. Give me a man with not goals and I'll give a stock clerk. - J. C. Penney

88. God heals, and the doctor takes the fee. - Benjamin Franklin

89. Great changes may not happen right away, but with effort even the difficult may become easy. - Bill Blackma

90. Great spirits have always encountered violent opposition from mediocre minds. - Albert Einstein

91. Gluttony is an emotional escape, a sign something is eating us. - Peter De Vries

92. Good humor is the health of the soul, sadness is its poison. - Lord Chesterfield

93. Having good health is very different from only being not sick. - Seneca The Younger

94. Happiness is nothing more than good health and a bad memory. - Albert Schweitzer

95. Happiness lies, first of all, in health. - George William Curtis

96. He cures most in whom most have faith. - Galen

97. He who has health has hope; and he who has hope has everything. - Arabic Proverb

98. Health is like money, we never have a true idea of its value until we lose it. - Josh Billings

99. Happiness is not something ready made. It comes from your own actions. - Dalai Lama
100. Happiness is when what you think, what you say, and what you do are in harmony. - Mohandas K Gandhi

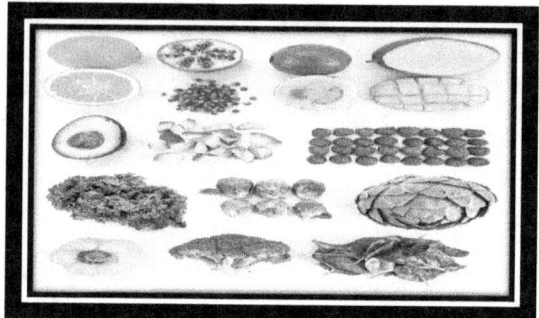

101.　　He said, 'If you listen carefully to the voice of the Lord your God and do what is right in His eyes, if you pay attention to His commands and keep all of His decrees, I will not bring on you any of the diseases I brought on the Egyptians, for I am the Lord, who heals you.' - Exodus 15:26

102.　　He who is not courageous enough to take risks will accomplish nothing in life. - Muhammad Ali

103.　　Health is not a condition of matter, but of Mind. - Mary Baker Eddy

104.　　Health is not valued till sickness comes. - Dr. Thomas Fuller

105.　　Health is the greatest gift, contentment the greatest wealth, faithfulness the best relationship. – Buddha

106. Health is the greatest possession. Contentment is the greatest treasure. Confidence is the greatest friend. Non-being is the greatest joy. - Lao Tzu

107. Holding on to anger is like holding on to a hot coal with the intent of throwing it at someone else; you are the one who gets burned. - Buddha

108. How do you live a long life? "Take a 2- mile walk every morning before breakfast." - Harry S. Truman

109. I am always doing that which I can not do, in order that I may learn how to do it. - Pablo Picasso

110. I am my own experiment. I am my own work of art. – Madonna

111. I am too positive to be doubtful, too optimistic to be fearful and too determined to be defeated. – Hussein Nishah

112. I believe that if you show people the problems and you show them the solutions they will be moved to act. - Bill Gates

113. I burned sixty calories. That should take care of a peanut I had in 1962. - Rita Rudner

114. I didn't start out about weight loss. I was very tired and my energy was low. This is my second go-around in love, so I want to make sure I'll be around to enjoy it. - Niecy Nash

115. I don't diet. I just don't eat as much as I'd like to. - Linda Evangelista

116. I don't know the key to success, but the key to failure is trying to please everybody. Bill Cosby

117. I don't want to hear excuses of why you can't; I want to hear reasons why you can. - Mr. Coker

118.     I failed my way to success. Thomas Edison

119.     I find the great thing in this world is not so much where we stand, as in what direction we are moving: To reach the port of heaven, we must sail sometimes with the wind and sometimes against it, but we must sail, and not drift, nor lie at anchor  - Oliver Wendell Holmes

120.     I found that people like rules, and I love to tell people what to do. It's not rocket science when it comes to weight loss. *It's about eating a little less and moving a little bit more. - Bob Harper*

121.     I freak out if I go a little too long without being in the gym. For a long time it was all about getting the weight off because I was 240 pounds at my heaviest, and now I'm around 175, so the majority of that weight loss was due to diet and exercise. - Nick Carter

122.     I have gained and lost the same ten pounds so many times over and over again my cellulite must have déjà vu. - Jane Wagner

123.     I have more energy to run after our four children. Weight loss and great skin were a bonus! - Niecy Nash

124.     I have not failed once. I've just found 10,000 ways that didn't work. Thomas Edison

125.     I have been impressed with the urgency of doing. Knowing is not enough; we must apply. Being willing is not enough; we must do. - Leonardo da Vinci

126.     I hear and I forget. I see and I remember. I do and I understand. – Confucius

127. I keep six honest serving men. They taught me all I knew. Their names are What and Why and When and How and Where and Who. - Rudyard Kipling

128. I keep trying to lose weight but it keeps finding me. – Anonymous

129. I look to the future because that's where I'm going to spend the rest of my life. - George Burns

130. I know a lot of men who are healthier at age fifty than they have ever been before, because a lot of their fear is gone. - Robert Bly

131. I never worry about diets. The only carrots that interest me are the number you get in a diamond. - Mae West

132. I see rejection in my skin, worry in my cancers, bitterness and hate in my aching joints. I failed to take care of my mind, and so my body now goes to hospital. - Astrid Alauda

133. I tried every diet in the book. I tried some that werent in the book. I tried eating the book. It tasted better than most of the diets. - Dolly Parton

134. I tried the Scarsdale diet and the Stillman water diet (you remember that one, where you run weight off trying to get to the bathroom). - Dolly Parton

135. I went on a diet, swore off drinking and heavy eating, and in fourteen days I had lost exactly two weeks. - Joe E. Lewis

136. If I had an hour to solve a problem, I'd spend 55 minutes thinking about the problem and 5 minutes thinking about solutions. - Albert Einstein

137. If I'd known I was going to live so long, I'd have taken better care of myself. - Leon Eldred

138. If I hired one of the stock boys to chase me around the store with a licorice whip, I'd be thin by Christmas. - Jennette Fulda

139. If I see a roadblock when I'm going down a highway, I don't wait for someone to build me a different highway. I find a different route. - Angela White

140. If we could give every individual the right amount of nourishment and exercise, not too little and not too much, we would have found the safest way to health. – Hippocrates

141. If we don't change we don't grow. If we don't grow, we are not really living. – Gail Sheehy

142. If you are working on something exciting that you really care about, you don't have to be pushed. The vision pulls you. - Steve Jobs

143. If you ask what is the single most important key to longevity, I would have to say it is avoiding worry, stress and tension. And if you didn't ask me, I'd still have to say it. - George Burns

144. If you are always trying to be normal, you will never know how amazing you can be. – Maya Angelou

145. If you care enough for the result, you will almost always attain it - William James

146. If you don't dare to begin, you don't stand a chance of getting there. - Anonymous

147. If you're tired of starting over, stop giving up.—Sparkpeople.com

148. If you believe that weight loss requires self-deprivation, I'm going to teach you otherwise. - Robert Atkins

149. If you don't do what's best for your body, you're the one who comes up on the short end. - Julius Erving

150. If you don't know where you are going how will you know when you get there? – Anonymous

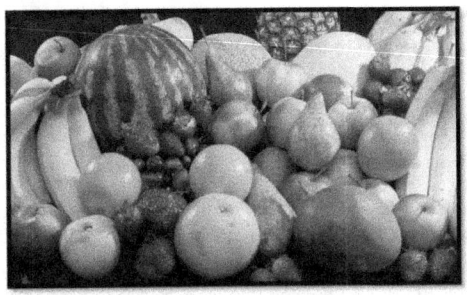

151. If you have health, you probably will be happy, and if you have health and happiness, you have all the wealth you need, even if it is not all you want. - Elbert Hubbard

152. If you keep on eating unhealthy food than no matter how many weight loss tips you follow, you are likely to retain weight and become obese. If only you start eating healthy food, you will be pleasantly surprised how easy it is to lose weight. - Subodh Gupt

153. If you think you are beaten you are, if you think you dare not, you don't. If you like to win, but you think you can't, it is almost certain you won't. - Napoleon Hill

154. If you want one year of prosperity, grow seeds. If you want ten years of prosperity, grow trees. If you want 100 years of prosperity, grow people. - Chinese Proverb

155. If you wish to grow thinner, diminish your dinner. – H. S. Leigh

156. If you worried about falling off the bike, you'd never get on. - Lance Armstrong

157. If your ship doesn't come in, swim out to it. - Jonathan Winters

158. I'm learning a lot about the culture of weight loss. I didn't know there were bloggers out there who were proud to be fat. - Mick Cornett

159. I'm not against working out. It's just not effective for weight loss. I like strength training to tone and firm the body so you look tight. But working out just makes you hungrier. - Jorge Cruise

160. I'm not overweight. I'm just nine inches too short. - Shelley Winters

161. I'm not overweight, I'm undertall. - Anonymous

162. I'm prouder of my weight loss than my Oscar! - Jennifer Hudson

163. Imagine the extraordinary. Be the extraordinary. -Garnet Hill

164. Instead of giving myself reasons why I can't, I give myself reasons why I can. – Anonymous

165. In all affairs it's a healthy thing now and then to hang a question mark on the things you have long taken for granted. - Bertrand Russell

166. In general, mankind, since the improvement of cookery, eat twice as much as nature requires. - Franklin

167. In order to succeed, your desire for success should be greater than your fear of failure. - Bill Cosby

168. In this age, which believes that there is a short cut to everything, the greatest lesson to be learned is that the most difficult way is, in the long run, the easiest! --Henry Miller

169. In this age, which believes that there is a short cut to everything, the greatest lesson to be learned is that the most difficult way is, in the long run, the easiest! --Henry Miller

170. Inaction breeds doubt and fear. Action breeds confidence and courage! - Dale Carnegie

171. It had dawned on me that the occurrence of a defect was the result of some condition or action, and that it would be possible to eliminate defects entirely by pursuing the cause. - Shigeo Shingo

172. It is time for us to stand and cheer for the doer, the achiever, the one who recognises the challenge and does something about it. - Vince Lombardi

173. It takes about four days of virtuous living to create a little weight loss. That also happens to be the time required to get used to eating less. In other words, if you can get past day three of a fitness regimen, things improve. - Martha Beck

174. Its not stress that kills us, it is our reaction to it. - Hans Selye

175. It's all about creating healthy habits rather than restrictions. – Anonymous

176. It's not what you do once in a while, It's what you do day in and day out that makes the difference. - Jenny Craig

177. It's not what you look like, that makes you who you are. It's what you do, that makes you who you are. Anonymous

178. ...It's true, the scale can only give you a numerical reflection of your relationship with gravity. That's it. It cannot measure beauty, talent, purpose, life force, possibility, strength, or love. Don't give the scale more power than it has earned. Take note of the number, then get off the scale and live your life. You are beautiful!" — Steve Maraboli

179. I've been absolutely terrified every moment of my life - and I've never let it keep me from doing a single thing I wanted to do. – Georgia O'Keeffe

180. I've been absolutely terrified every moment of my life - and I've never let it keep me from doing a single thing I wanted to do. – Georgia O'Keeffe

181. I've failed over and over and over again in my life and that is why I succeed. - Michael Jordan

182. Junk food you've craved for an hour, or the body you've craved for a lifetime? Your decision. – Anonymous

183. Keep away from people who try to belittle your ambitions. Small people always do that, but the really great make you feel that you, too, can become great. Mark Twain

184. Keep your face to the sunshine and you can not see the shadows. - Helen Keller

185. Learn to love yourself. If you say "I accept myself unconditionally right now" twice a day for 30 days, by day 28 you will be believing it! - Anonymous

186. Learning is the beginning of wealth. Learning is the beginning of health. Learning is the beginning of spirituality. Searching and learning is where the miracle process all begins. - Jim Rohn

187. Leave your drugs in the chemist's pot if you can cure the patient with food. - Hippocrates

188.    Let thy food be thy medicine and thy medicine be thy food. – Hippocrates

189.    Live in rooms full of light. Avoid heavy food. Be moderate in the drinking of wine. Take massage, baths, exercise, and gymnastics. Fight insomnia with gentle rocking or the sound of running water Change surroundings and take long journeys. Strictly avoid frightening ideas. Indulge in cheerful conversation and amusements. Listen to music. - A. Cornelius Celsus

190.    Log off. Shut down. Go run. -Women's Running

191.    Love yourself first and everything else falls into line. – Lucille Ball

192.    Man can put out about $1/20^{th}$ of a horsepower. He has to rest at least 9 hours a day. He also has to eat and drink. As a power source, we are terrible. However, it is when man starts thinking of ideas that the difference between man and machine emerges. - Soichiro Honda

193.    Man will put up with any "how" if he has a "why. - Friedrich Wilhelm Nietzsche

194.    Marathon runners don't worry about the conditions, they just run anyway! – Anonymous

195.    Medicine is a collection of uncertain prescriptions, the results of which taken collectively, are more fatal than useful to mankind. Water, air and cleanliness are the chief articles in my pharmacopeia. - Napoleon Bonaparte

196.    Medicine is an advancing science and the best hospitals in the world are not those which merely use new technology but those which create it. - Sir George Pickering

197.    Men succeed when they realize that their failures are the preparation for their victories. - Ralph Waldo Emerson

198. Mental health is defined as a state of well-being in which every individual realizes his or her own potential, can cope with the normal stresses of life, can work productively and fruitfully, and is able to make a contribution to her or his community. —World Health Organization, 2014

199. Most diseases are the result of medication which has been prescribed to relieve and take away a beneficient and warning symptom on the part of Nature. - Elbert Hubbard

200. Most weight loss diets center around portion control, which is just trying to eat smaller amounts of the same addictive foods. This approach inevitably fails. - Joel Fuhrman

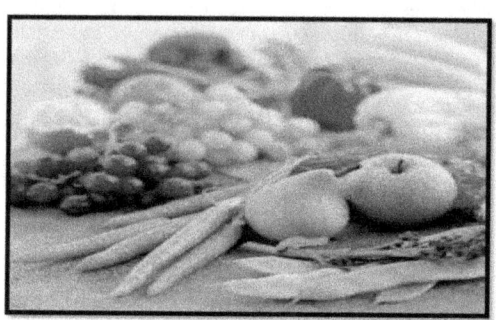

201.    Most people spend more time and energy going around problems than trying to solve them. - Henry Ford

202.    Motivation is what gets you started. Habit is what keeps you going. – Jim Ryan

203.    Movement is a medicine for creating change in person's physical, emotional, and mental states. – Carol Welch

204.    My doctor told me to stop having intimate dinners for four. Unless there are three other people. - Orson Welles

205.    My success has been something I've worked a long time at and it's been a gradual process. I compare it to the idea of someone losing a lot of weight over a period of a few years. You don't really notice the weight loss overall but if you compare photos from then and now there's a big difference. - Ray William Johnson

206.    Nature, time and patience are three great physicians. - H.G. Bohn

207.    Never eat more than you can lift. - Miss Piggy

208.    Never give in, never give in, never, never, never never in nothing, great or small, large or petty never give in except to convictions of honor and good sense.- Winston Churchill

209.    Never, never, never, never give up. - Winston Churchill

210. No, as it turns out, I really like being congratulated on my weight loss. I like it so much, it's tragic. - Carrie Fisher

211. No diet will remove all the fat from your body because the brain is entirely fat. Without a brain, you might look good, but all you could do is run for public office. - George Bernard Shaw

212. No Illness which can be treated by the diet should be treated by any other means. - Moses Maimonides

213. No problem can be solved from the same level of consciousness that created it. - Albert Einstein

214. Not-knowing is true knowledge. Presuming to know is a disease First realize that you are sick; then you can move toward health - Lao Tzu

215. Nothing tastes as good as being thin feels. - Elizabeth Berg

216. Obstacles are what we see when we take our eyes off the goal. - Rita Davenport

217. On need of supplement & vitamins- "If you eat a balanced diet you get all the vitamins and minerals you need and you don't need any supplement and overdosing can actually be more harmful." - Subodh Gupta

218. One can not think well, love well or sleep well if one has not dined well. - Virginia Woolf

219. One meal a day is enough for a lion and it ought to be for a man. - G. Fordyce

220. One meal a day is enough for a lion and would be for all of us if all we did all day was swat flies. - Erma Bombeck

221. One of the first duties of the physician is to educate the masses not to take medicine. - William Osler

222. One should eat to live, not live to eat. - Anonymous

223. Only those who risk going too far can possibly find out how far one can go... -T.S. Eliot

224. Optimism is the one quality more associated with success and happiness than any other. - Robert F Kennedy

225. "Or do you not know that your body is the temple of the Holy Spirit who is in you, whom you have from God, and you are not your own? For you were bought at a price; therefore glorify God in your body and in your spirit, which are God's." - 1 Corinthians 6:19-20

226. Our greatest glory is not in never falling, but in rising ever time we fall – Confucius

227. Pain is inevitable. Suffering is optional. - M. Kathleen Casey

228. Pain is temporary. Quitting lasts forever. - Lance Armstrong

229. Part of the secret of success in life is to eat what you like and let the food fight it out inside. - Mark Twain

230. People say that losing weight is no walk in the park. When I hear that I think, yeah, that's the problem. – Chris Adams

231. People support what they create. - Kurt Lewin

232. Perfection is not attainable, but if we chase perfection we can catch excellence. - Vince Lombardi

233. Perseverance is the secret of all triumphs. Victor Hugo

234. Pleasant words are like a honeycomb, Sweetness to the soul and health to the bones. – Proverbs 16:4

235. Push yourself. Because no one else is going to do it for you. - Anonymous

236. Reality check: you can never, ever, use weight loss to solve problems that are not related to your weight. At your goal weight or not, you still have to live with yourself and deal with your problems. You will still have the same husband, the same job, the same kids, and the same life. Losing weight is not a cure for life. - Phillip C. McGraw

237. Rest, as soon as there is pain, is a great restorative in all disturbances of the body. - Hippocrates

238. Rule your mind or it will rule you. – Horace

239. Slipping backwards? You may be backing up to get a running start. – Dan Millman

240. Simple diet is best; for many dishes bring many diseases; and rich sauces are worse than heaping several meats upon each other. - Pliny

241. Sleep is the best meditation. - Dalai Lama

242. So many people spend their health gaining wealth, and then have to spend their wealth to regain their health. - A.J. Reb Materi

243. ...So while you may not be able to change the wiring in your brain, you can "feed" those reward centers other pleasures...Biology isn't destiny when you have effective strategies... - Bob Greene

244. Self-love is the only weight-loss aid that really works in the long run. - Jenny Craig

245. Some people want it to happen; some wish it would happen; others make it happen. - Michael Jordan

246. Some people think that doctors and nurses can put scrambled eggs back into the shell. - Dorothy Canfield Fisher

247. Some succeed because they are destined to, but most succeed because they are determined to. - G. Clegg

248. Start by doing what's necessary; then do what's possible; and suddenly you are doing the impossible. - Saint Francis of Assisi

249. Start Today Not Tomorrow - Anonymous

250. Strive for progress, not perfection. –Unknown

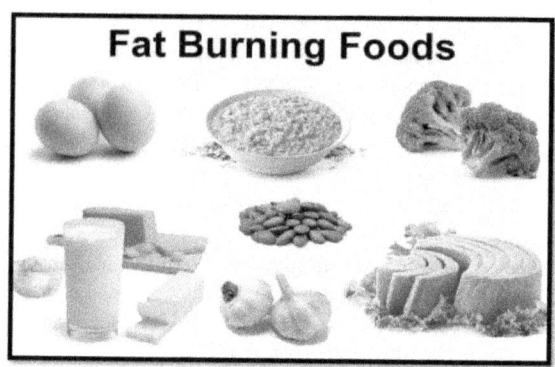

**Fat Burning Foods**

251.     Stumbling is not falling. - Portuguese Proverb

252.     Success is not a place that we aspire to, it is a process in which we live by. Often the only ingredient being the ability to not quit – Anonymous

253.     Success seems to be connected to action. Successful people keep moving. They make mistakes, but they don't quit. - Conrad Hilton

254.     Successful weight loss takes programming, not willpower. - Phil McGraw

255.     Sustainable weight loss is a complete lifestyle change, not a 12 week eating plan. – Anonymous

256.     Take care of your body. It's the only place you have to live. - Jim Rohn

257. Tell me, I forget. Teach me, I learn. Involve me, I remember. Ben Franklin

258. Thank you for calling the Weight Loss Hotline. If you'd like to lose a half pound right now, press 1 eighteen thousand times. – Randy Glasbergen

259. That which we persist in doing becomes easier to do; not that the nature of the thing itself is changed, but that our power to do is increased. - Ralph Waldo Emerson

260. The 2nd day of a diet is always easier than the 1st. By the 2nd day you're off it. - Jackie Gleason

261. The art of medicine consists of amusing the patient while nature cures the disease. - Voltaire

262. The belly is ungrateful--it always forgets we already gave it something. - Russian Proverb

263. The best exercise is pushing yourself away from the table. - Grandpa Arthur Strutz

264. The best way to get something done is to begin. – Anonymous

265. The best way to have a good idea is to have lots of ideas. - Linus Pauling

266. The best way to lose weight is to eat all you want of everything you don't like. – Anonymous

267. The biggest disease today is not leprosy or tuberculosis, but rather the feeling of being unwanted. - Mother Theresa

268. The biggest weight loss secret? Manage your emotions or they will keep mismanaging you. - Brian Vaszily

269. The difference between who you are and who you want to be is what you do. - Anonymous

270. The fishermen know the sea is dangerous and the storms are terrible, but they have never found this sufficient reason to remain on shore." Vincent Van Gogh

271. The first wealth is health. - Ralph Waldo Emerson

272. The goal in life is living in agreement with nature. – Zeno

273. The good Lord gave you a body that can stand most anything. It's your mind you have to convince. - Vince Lombardi

274. The greatest discovery of any generation is that human beings can alter their lives by altering the attitudes of their minds." Dr. Albert Schweitzer

275. The greatest of follies is to sacrifice health for any other kind of happiness. – Arthur Schopenhauer

276. The greatest mistake you can make in life is to be continually fearing you will make one. Elbert Hubbard

277. The greatest source of competitive advantage is not really cost or quality, but creativity. - John Micklethwait

278. The greatest wealth is health. - Virgil

279. The groundwork of all happiness is health. - Leigh Hunt

280. The human body was designed to walk, run or stop; it wasn't built for coasting. - Cullen Hightower

281. The fastest way to lose weight is to find religion and start fasting. - Jarod Kintz

282. The foods that are recommended today are as palatable as a steady diet of wet blotters. - Groucho Marx

283. The greatest mistake you can make in life is to be continually fearing you will make one. - Elbert Hubbard

284. The improvement of understanding is for two ends: first, our own increase of knowledge; secondly, to enable us to deliver that knowledge to others. - John Locke

285. The man who can drive himself further once the effort gets painful is the man who will win. - Roger Bannister

286. The man who fears suffering is already suffering from what he fears. - Michel De Montaigne

287. The minute you settle for less than you deserve, you get even less than you settled for. - Maureen Dowd

288. The more serious the illness, the more important it is for you to fight back, mobilizing all your resources - spiritual, emotional, intellectual, and physical. - Normin Cousins

289. The next major advance in the health of the American people will be determined by what the individual is willing to do for himself." - John Knowles

290. The odds of hitting a target go up dramatically when you aim at it. – Mal Pancoast

291. The only cure for grief is action. - George Henry Lewis


292. The older you get, the tougher it is to lose weight because by then, your body and your fat are really good friends - Anonymos

293. The only way to keep your health is to eat what you don't want, drink what you don't like and do what you'd rather not. - Mark Twain

294. The... patient should be made to understand that he or she must take charge of his own life. Don't take your body to the doctor as if he were a repair shop. - Quentin Regestein

295. The price of success is much lower than the price of failure. - Zig Ziglar

296. The problem isn't people eating too much, but rather people not burning off enough calories. - Daniel L. Worona

297. The processes of disease aim not at the destruction of life, but the saving of it. - Frederick

298. The quality, not the longevity, of one's life is what is important. - Martin Luther King, Jr.


299. The reason most people never reach their goals is that they don't define them, or ever seriously consider them as believable or achievable. Winners can tell you where they are going, what they plan to do along the way, and who will be sharing the adventure with them. - Dennis Waitley

300.     The reasonable man adapts himself to the world; the unreasonable man persists in trying to adapt the world to himself. Therefore all progress depends on the unreasonable man. - George Bernard Shaw

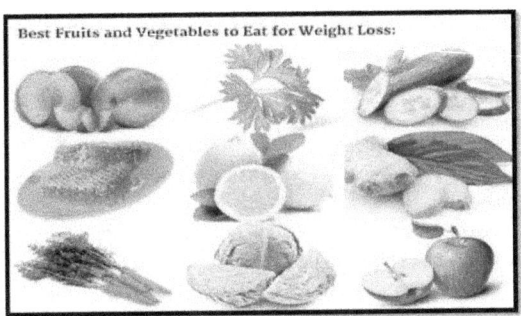

Best Fruits and Vegetables to Eat for Weight Loss:

301. The rest of the world lives to eat, while I eat to live. – Socrates

302. The road to someday, leads to the town of nowhere. Procrastination is the silent killer. - Anthony Robbins

303. The real pride, the real present, is your health and your longevity. My whole career, I have never done anything where competition was involved with weight loss. - Richard Simmons

304. The road to someday, leads to the town of nowhere. Procrastination is the silent killer. - Anthony Robbins

305. The safest thing for a patient is to be in the hands of a man engaged in teaching medicine. In order to be a teacher of medicine the doctor must always be a student. - Charles H. Mayo

306. The scientific truth may be put quite briefly; eat moderately, having an ordinary mixed diet, and don't worry. - Robert Hutchison

307. The secret of getting ahead is getting started. The secret of getting started is breaking your complex overwhelming tasks into small manageable tasks, and then starting on the first one. Mark Twain

308. The secret of health for both mind and body is not to mourn for the past, worry about the future, or anticipate troubles, but to live in the present moment wisely and earnestly. - Buddha

309. The secret to getting ahead is getting started. - Mark Twain

310. The time for action is now. It's never too late to do something. - Carl Sandburg

311. The seeds of great discoveries are constantly floating around, but they only take root in minds well prepared to receive them. - Joseph Henry

312. The time for action is now. It's never too late to do something. - Carl Sandburg

313. The treatments themselves do not 'cure' the condition, they simply restore the body's self-healing ability. - Leon Chaitow

314. The tragedy in life doesn't lie in not reaching your goal. The tragedy lies in having no goal to reach. - Benjamin Mays

315. The trouble about always trying to preserve the health of the body is that it is so difficult to do without destroying the health of the mind. - G. K. Chesterton

316. The trouble with the rat race is that even if you win you're still a rat. Lily Tomlin

317. The typical old-fashioned diet (in the nineteenth century) was so bad it almost assembled modern dieting. - P. J. O'Rourke

318. The ultimate measure of a man is not where he stands in moments of comfort and convenience, but where he stands at times of challenge and controversy. - Martin Luther King, Jr

319. The way you think, the way you behave, the way you eat, can influence your life by 30 to 50 years. - Deepak Chopra

320. The world of achievement has always belonged to the optimist. - Harold Wilkins

321. There are no big problems, there are just a lot of little problems. - Henry Ford

322. There are no such things as incurables, there are only things for which man has not found a cure. - Bernard Baruch

323. There are some remedies worse than the disease. - Publius Syrus

324. There are two choices really. You can either surrender to the pressures of life and the struggles of this particular battle.... or you continue the fight...and do so with even more vengence and determination to reach your goals then you did before. I choose the fight.....I know what it will get me. – Kim (Getting2Goal.com)

325. There are two primary choices in life; to accept conditions as they exist, or accept the responsibility for changing them. - Denis Waitley

326. There are many ways of going forward, but only one way of standing still. - Franklin D. Roosevelt

327. There are many ways to fail, but only one way to succeed; NEVER GIVE UP! - J. Pangalila

328. There are two great medicines: Diet and Self-Control. - Max Bircher

329. There are two ways of meeting difficulties, you alter the difficulties or you alter yourself to meet them.- Phyllis Bottome

330. There is no diet that will do what eating healthy does. – Anonymous

331. There - is no fate that plans men's lives. Whatever comes to us, good or bad, is usually the result of our own action or lack of action. - Herbert N. Casson

332. There is no need to worry about mere size. We do not necessarily respect a fat man more than a thin man. Sir Isaac Newton was very much smaller than a hippopotamus, but we do not on that account value him less. - Bertrand Russell

333. There is no one giant step that does it. It's a lot of little steps. - Peter A. Cohen

334. There is no such thing as luck. Success comes from actually doing it. – Anonymous

335. There is nothing permanent except change. – Heraclitus

336. They are as sick that surfeit with too much, as they that starve with nothing. - Shakespeare

337.    Those who cannot change their minds cannot change anything. - George Bernard Shaw

338.    Those who think they have no time for healthy eating will sooner or later have to find time for illness. – Anonymous

339.    Those who wish to sing, always find a song. - Swedish Proverb

340.    To accomplish great things, we must not only act, but also dream; not only plan, but also believe. - Anatole France

341.    To avoid sickness eat less; to prolong life worry less. - Chu Hui Weng

342.    To keep the body in good health is a duty, otherwise we shall not be able to keep our mind strong and clear. – Buddha

343.    To wish to be well is a part of becoming well. - Seneca

344.    Transformation literally means going beyond your form. – Wayne Dyer

345.    Ultimately, the only power to which man should aspire is that which he exercises over himself. - Elie Wiesel

346.    Unhealthy places and decadent times infect us by their contagion. - Joubert

347.    Unless you try to do something beyond what you have already mastered, you will never grow. - Ronald E. Osborn

348. Victory is always possible for the person who refuses to stop fighting.
– Napoleon Hill

349. We all have dreams. But in order to make dreams come into reality, it takes an awful lot of determination, dedication, self-discipline, and effort.
- Jesse Owens

350. We are healed of a suffering only by experiencing it to the full. -
Marcel Proust

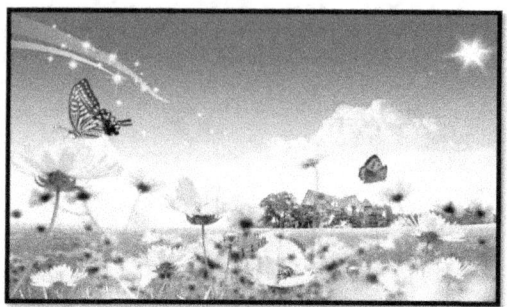

351.  We are more apt to catch the vices of others than their virtues, as disease is far more contagious than health. - Charles Caleb Colton

352.  We are what we repeatedly do, excellence, therefore, is not an act but a habit. – Aristotle

353.  We cannot seek or attain health, wealth, learning, justice or kindness in general. Action is always specific, concrete, individualized, unique. - Benjamin Jowett

354.  We define innovation as the successful implementation of creative ideas within an organization. - Theresa Amabile

355.  We forget ourselves and our destinies in health, and the chief use of temporary sickness is to remind us of these concerns. - Ralph Waldo Emerson

356.  We must accept finite disappointment, but we must never lose infinite hope. - Dr Martin Luther King Jr.

357.  We must become the change we want to see. - Gandhi

358.  We never repent of having eaten too little. - Thomas Jefferson

359.    We should always presume the disease to be curable, until its own nature prove it otherwise. - Peter Mere Latham

360.    Weight loss can change your whole character. That always amazed me: Shedding pounds does change your personality. It changes your philosophy of life because you recognize that you are capable of using your mind to change your body. - Jean Nidetch

361.    Weight loss is not the key to your dreams. The truth is there is no lock and the door is flimsy. - Golda Poretsky

362.    Well done is better than well said. - Ben Franklin

363.    What people say, what people do, and what they say they do are entirely different things. - Margaret Meade

364.    What you eat standing up doesn't count - Beth Barnes

365.    When a man is laboring under the pain of any distemper, it is then that he recollects there is a God, and that he himself is but a man. - Pliny

366.    When I started working out, it wasn't about weight loss; I was going through a really hard time and needed an emotional release. Once you start getting in the tabloids claiming you have fake body parts, then it's like, 'Okay, I made it. Now I'm really working out. - Khloe Kardashian

367.    When it comes to eating right and exercising, there is no "I'll start tomorrow. "Tomorrow is disease." – Terri Guillements

368.    "When one approach is not working to reach the desired goal, that's not a reason to abandon the goal. Instead, it is time to devise another approach."------Ralph Marston

369.     When one door closes another door opens; but we so often look so long and so regretfully upon the closed door, that we do not see the ones which open for us. - Alexander Graham Bell

370.     When one door of happiness closes, another opens; but often we look so long at the closed door that we do not see the one which has been opened for us. - Helen Keller

371.     When people tell me they can't afford to join a gym, I tell them to go outside; planet Earth is a gym and we're already members. Run, climb, sweat, and enjoy all of the natural wonder that is available to you. - Steve Maraboli

372.     When the patient loves his disease, how unwilling he is to allow a remedy to be applied. - Pierre Corneille

373.     When the sun comes up each day, be up and out with it. – Anonymous

374.     When the world says, Give up, Hope whispers, Try it one more time. Anonymous

375.     When we are well, we all have good advice for those who are ill. - Terrence

376.     When you get into a tight place and everything goes against you, till it seems as though you could not hold on a minute longer, never give up then, for that is just the place and time that the tide will turn. - Harriet Beecher Stowe

377.     When your body absorbs toxins, it stores them in fat, which is why fiber and probiotics are strategic weapons for weight loss. Fiber keeps your colon healthy and reduces your body's absorption of toxins. - Suzanne Somers

378. Whether you think that you can, or that you can't, you are usually right. - Henry Ford

379. While weight loss is important, what's more important is the quality of food you put in your body - food is information that quickly changes your metabolism and genes. - Mark Hyman

380. Winners feel like winners Losers feel like losers How do you feel? – Anonymous

381. Without health, life is not life; it is only a state of languor and suffering. - Francois Rabelais

382. Who of you by worrying can add a single hour to his life? Since you can not do this very little thing, why do you worry about the rest?" - Luke 12:25-26

383. Worrying does not empty tomorrow of its troubles; it empties today of its strength. – Anonymous

384. Yesterday is gone. Tomorrow has not yet come. We have only today. Let us begin. - Mother Teresa

385. You are as important to your health as it is to you. – Terri Guillemets

386. You are far too smart to be the only thing standing in your way. – Jennifer Freeman

387. You are the sole genuine obstacle in your path to a fulfilling lifestyle. - Les Brown

388. You can either hold yourself up to the unrealistic standards of others, or ignore them and concentrate on being happy with yourself as you are. - J. Jacques

389. You can feel sore tomorrow or you can feel sorry tomorrow. You choose. – Anonymous

390. You can turn painful situations around through laughter. If you can find humor in anything, even poverty, you can survive it. - Bill Cosby

391. You can't be a winner and be afraid to lose. - Charles Lynch

392. You can't learn how to ride a bike by reading a book on physics. - Anonymous

393. You can't start the next chapter of your life if you keep rereading the last one. - Anonymous

394. You don't have to be great to start, but you have to start to be great. – Anonymous

395. You don't understand anything until you learn it more than one way. Marvin Minsky

396. You have a choice. You can throw in the towel, or you can use it to wipe the sweat off your face. - Anonymous

397. You have failed only when you quit trying. Until then, you're still in the act of progression. So, never quit trying and you'll never be a failure.--- Tommy Kelley

398. You have to stay in shape. My grandmother, she started walking five miles a day when she was 60. She's 97 today and we don't know where the hell she is. - Ellen Degeneres

399. You have to manage a system. The system doesn't manage itself. - W. Edwards Deming, Ph.D.

400. You miss 100% of the shots you never take. - Wayne Gretzky

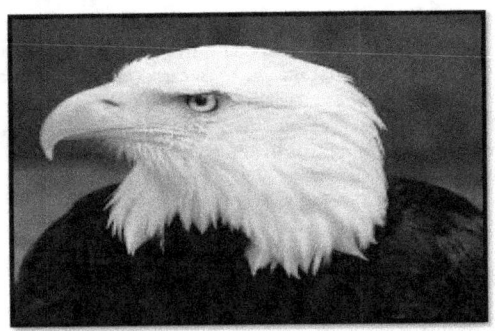

401. You've only got 3 choices in life: Give up, give in, or give it all you've got. – Anonymous

402. You may be disappointed if you fail, but you are doomed if you don't try. - Beverly Sills

403. You will never be happier than you expect. To change your happiness, change your expectation. - Bette Davis

404. You will never know your limits unless you push yourself to them. - Anonymous

405. You know what the secret to weight loss is? Don't eat much. - Simon Cowell

406. You must act as if it is impossible to fail. - Ashanti Proverb

407. You need to know what you are eating, how much you're eating and how many calories that food has to be successful at weight loss. – Dr McTiernan

408. You must begin to think of yourself as becoming the person you want to be. - David Viscott

409. Your body is a reflection of what you are. If you want to look healthy, you will have to be healthy. - Anonymous

410. Your body is the baggage you must carry through life. The more excess the baggage, the shorter the trip. - Anonymous

411.	Your desire to change must be greater than your desire to stay the same. - Anonymous

412.	Your body is the baggage you must carry through life. The more excess the baggage, the shorter the trip. - Arnold H. Glasgow

413.	Your goals, minus your doubts, equal your reality. - Ralph Marston

414.	Your life is not a rehearsal. Don't leave it without giving it your all. – Anonymous

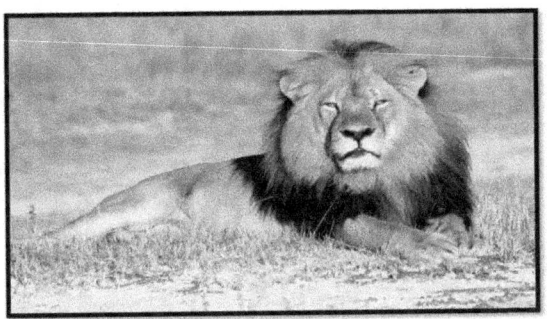

415. Don't Quit

When you've eaten too much and you can't write it down, And you feel like the biggest failure in town. When you want to give up just because you gave in, and forget all about being healthy and thin. So What! You went over your points a bit, It's your next move that counts...So don't you quit! It's a moment of truth, it's an attitude change. It's learning the skills to get back in your range. It's telling yourself, "You've done great up till now. You can take on this challenge and beat it somehow." It's part of your journey toward reaching your goal. You're still gonna make it, just stay in control. To stumble and fall is not a disgrace, If you summon the will to get back in the race. But, often the struggler's, when loosing their grip, Just throw in the towel and continue to slip. And learn too late when the damage is done, that the race wasn't over...they still could have won. Lifestyle change can be awkward and slow, but facing each challenge will help you grow. Success is failure turned inside out, the silver tint in a cloud of doubt. When you're pushing to the brink, just refuse to submit, If you bite it, you write it....But don't you quit! – Anonymous

Thanks for reading through this mini book and I am absolutely sure you have discovered at least one or more nuggets which had made deep impression on you; if adequately applied I am certain will bring a positive change in you!

I wish you the best!!

Timothy J.

tim4real20@gmail.com

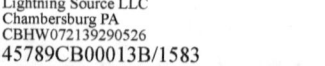